Dr. Macklene. C. Jones

THE PROSTATE CANCER GUIDEBOOK

Understanding symptoms, treatment options and prevention strategies

<u>5</u>

CONCLUSION

INTRODUCTION

Prostate cancer is a major public health concern for men worldwide. One in every eight men will be diagnosed with prostate cancer during their lifetime, according to estimates. While prostate cancer is a serious and potentially fatal condition, there is still hope. Many men with prostate cancer can live long and healthy lives if it is detected early and treated appropriately.

This book's goal is to be a thorough guide to understanding prostate cancer. Whether you or a loved one has been diagnosed with prostate cancer, or you are simply curious about the disease, this book will give you the information you need to make informed health decisions.

This book will go over a wide range of prostate cancer-related issues, such as the structure of the prostate gland, the numerous forms of prostate cancer, typical symptoms and signs of the disease, and the various diagnostic tests and procedures used to diagnose prostate cancer.

We will also go over the various prostate cancer treatment choices, such as surgery, radiation therapy, hormone therapy, and chemotherapy. We will also look at several complementary and alternative medicines that are sometimes used to treat prostate cancer.

Living with prostate cancer can be difficult, and we will provide practical guidance on how to cope with a diagnosis, manage treatment side effects, and locate support for sufferers and their families. We will also talk about lifestyle adjustments that can help lower the chance of developing prostate cancer or improve the results of individuals who have already been diagnosed.

Finally, we will examine the most recent achievements in prostate cancer research, including novel therapies and preventative techniques, and provide advice on how to stay current with the field's latest developments.

This book is a useful resource that will help you navigate the complex and often perplexing world of prostate cancer, whether you are facing a diagnosis or simply want to learn more about this important health issue. You can take control of your health and make informed decisions that will help you live a long and healthy life by arming yourself with knowledge and insight.

1

WHAT EXACTLY IS PROSTATE CANCER?

Prostate cancer is a form of cancer that develops in the prostate gland, which is a tiny gland in males found directly below the bladder. The prostate gland is an important aspect of the male reproductive system because it generates a fluid that helps nurture and transport sperm. Prostate cancer is one of the most frequent cancers among men, with a projected 248,530 new cases and 34,130 deaths in the United States alone in 2021.

Prostate Cancer Risk Factors

Prostate cancer has various risk factors, including age, family history, and race. Prostate cancer is most typically diagnosed in males over the age of 50, and the risk of having it rises with age. Men who have a family history of prostate cancer, especially if it occurred in a close relative such as a father or brother, are also at a higher risk of having the disease. Furthermore, men of African American heritage have a higher risk of developing prostate cancer than men of other races and ethnicities.

WHAT ARE THE PROSTATE CANCER STATISTICS AND RISK FACTORS?

Prostate cancer is one of the most frequent cancers among men globally, and its prevalence rises with age. The following are some major statistics and risk factors for prostate cancer:

Prostate cancer is the second largest cause of cancer death in males in the United States, after lung cancer, according to the American Cancer Society. An estimated 248,530 new instances of prostate cancer will be detected in 2021, with 34,130 men dying from the condition.

The incidence of prostate cancer varies greatly by race and ethnicity. African American males had the greatest incidence rate of prostate cancer in the United States, followed by non-Hispanic white men. Men of Hispanic and Asian/Pacific Islander origin have lower incidence rates.

Age is a significant risk factor for prostate cancer. The condition is uncommon in men under the age of 40, but the risk grows dramatically after the age of 50, with the majority of cases diagnosed in men over the age of 65.

Prostate cancer risk can also be increased by genetic alterations. Mutations in some genes, such as BRCA1 and BRCA2, have been associated with an increased risk of prostate cancer, as well as breast and Cancer of the ovaries.

Lifestyle factors may also play a role in the risk of prostate cancer. A diet high in red meat and dairy products and low in fruits and vegetables, according to some research, may raise the risk of prostate cancer. Other risk factors, such as obesity and smoking, may also be linked to an increased risk.

It is critical to understand that having one or more risk factors for prostate cancer does not guarantee that a man will get the disease. Many men who have one or more risk factors never acquire prostate cancer, but some men who have no known risk factors do. However, being aware of risk factors and taking actions to eliminate them, such as through lifestyle changes or frequent physical activity, can help lower the overall risk.

2

SYMPTOMS, DIAGNOSIS, AND STAGING

Prostate cancer is a disease that can present with a variety of symptoms, be detected using a variety of methods, and be staged according to severity and spread. This chapter will go over the signs of prostate cancer, the various techniques of diagnosis, and the different phases of the disease.

Prostate Cancer Symptoms

Because early-stage prostate cancer may not create any visible symptoms, frequent screening is critical for early identification. However, as the cancer progresses, it can cause a variety of symptoms, such as:

- **Urinary symptoms**: Increased frequency or urgency, difficulty starting or stopping urination, poor urine flow, and pain or burning when urinating.
- **Urine containing blood or sperm**
- Symptoms of pelvic pain or discomfort area, the lower back, or the hips
- Sexual dysfunction
- Appetite loss and weight loss
- Fatigue

It is crucial to remember that these symptoms can also be caused by other disorders, so a proper diagnosis from a healthcare professional is required.

PROSTATE CANCER DIAGNOSIS

Prostate cancer can be detected using a variety of approaches, including:

- A healthcare clinician performs a digital rectal exam (DRE) by inserting a gloved, lubricated finger into the rectum to feel for any abnormalities in the prostate gland.

- PSA (prostate-specific antigen) test: This blood test detects PSA, a protein generated by the prostate gland. PSA levels that are elevated can be a symptom of prostate cancer or other prostate disorders.

If an anomaly is discovered during a DRE or PSA, a biopsy is performed. A biopsy may be recommended as a test. A little tissue sample is extracted from the prostate gland and inspected under a microscope for cancer cells during this surgery.

PROSTATE CANCER STAGING

The number and extent of the malignant cells, as well as how far they have gone beyond the prostate gland, are used to stage prostate cancer. The stages of prostate cancer are as follows:

Stage I: The cancer is localized to the prostate gland and has not progressed to other parts of the body.

Stage II: The cancer is still contained within the prostate gland, but it has expanded in size and may have spread to adjacent tissues.

Stage III: The disease has gone beyond the prostate gland and may have infiltrated adjacent lymph nodes.

Stage IV: Other regions of the body, such as the bones, lungs, or liver, have been affected by the malignancy.

Knowing the stage of prostate cancer is critical for choosing the best treatment approach and forecasting the disease's fate.

Because the signs of prostate cancer may be undetectable in the early stages, regular screenings are critical for early detection. DRE, PSA testing, and biopsies can all be used to diagnose prostate cancer. The staging of prostate cancer is critical in selecting the best treatment approach and predicting the disease's fate

3

TREATMENT OPTIONS

Active Surveillance and Watchful Waiting

Active surveillance and watchful waiting are two prostate cancer management approaches that may be suggested for patients with low-risk or early-stage prostate cancer. These choices are usually considered for patients with a life expectancy of fewer than ten years or who have medical issues that make surgery or radiation therapy too dangerous.

Here are some examples of active surveillance and watchful waiting:

- Active surveillance entails closely monitoring prostate cancer with regular PSA blood tests, digital rectal exams, and sometimes biopsies.

- The purpose of active surveillance is to postpone or prevent therapy while closely monitoring the growth of the malignancy.

- If the cancer spreads or becomes more aggressive, treatments such as surgery or radiation therapy may be considered.

- Active surveillance is usually advised for people with low-risk prostate cancer, which means the tumor is tiny, restricted to the prostate gland, and progressing slowly.

- Active surveillance is comparable to watchful waiting, except it entails monitoring cancer without any active interventions.

This means that the patient is not receiving any therapies or biopsies and is instead being observed for cancer signs and changes. Patients with a restricted life expectancy or other major health issues that make therapy too risky are often advised to use watchful waiting.

Both active surveillance and watchful waiting have benefits and drawbacks. These procedures have the advantage of avoiding needless treatments and adverse effects associated with surgery or radiation therapy. Nonetheless, if left untreated for too long, the cancer may develop and become more difficult to treat.

Patients should examine the benefits and drawbacks of active surveillance versus watchful waiting with their healthcare physician before making an informed decision based on their unique circumstances. Regular check-ins with healthcare specialists are also necessary to monitor any changes in cancer and adapt the treatment strategy as needed.

RADIATION THERAPY AND SURGERY

Prostate cancer treatment options widely employed include surgery and radiation therapy. Both therapies are designed to eliminate or destroy cancer cells in the prostate gland and adjacent tissues. Here's a deeper look at each alternative:

Prostate cancer surgery entails removing the entire prostate gland as well as any adjacent lymph nodes and tissues that may be impacted by cancer. This is usually accomplished through either open surgery or minimally invasive surgery such as laparoscopic or robotic-assisted surgery. The purpose of surgery is to remove malignant tissue while also preventing cancer from spreading to other parts of the body. Patients with localized or early-stage prostate cancer are usually advised to undergo surgery.

Urinary incontinence, sexual dysfunction, and bowel issues are all possible adverse effects of prostate cancer surgery. However, developments in surgical methods have lowered the likelihood of severe complications. Patients should discuss the potential risks and advantages of surgery with their healthcare professional, as well as ask any questions they may have.

Radiation Treatment: Radiation treatment employs high-energy radiation beams to treat patients by eliminating cancer cells in the prostate gland. Radiation therapy can be administered either externally via a machine that focuses radiation beams on the prostate gland or internally by small radioactive pellets known as brachytherapy that are put inside the prostate gland. Patients with localized or early-stage prostate cancer are usually advised to undergo radiation therapy.

Radiation therapy may result in weariness, skin irritation, and urinary or gastrointestinal issues. However, these side effects usually go away within a few weeks to months of finishing treatment. Radiation therapy may be used with hormone therapy in some circumstances to improve outcomes.

As with surgery, patients should discuss the potential risks and advantages of radiation therapy with their healthcare provider and ask any questions they may have.

have.

Surgery and radiation therapy are both effective treatments for prostate cancer. The treatment chosen will be determined by various criteria, including the stage and grade of cancer, the patient's overall health, and their personal preferences. Patients must collaborate closely with their healthcare professionals to build a personalized treatment plan that matches their specific needs.

HORMONE REPLACEMENT TREATMENT

Hormone therapy, also known as **androgen deprivation therapy (ADT)**, is a prostate cancer treatment strategy that tries to reduce the number of male hormones in the body, mainly testosterone. Because prostate cancer cells rely on male hormones to thrive and spread, hormone therapy can reduce or stop the growth of prostate cancer.

Hormone treatment entails the use of drugs, which can be given in a variety of ways, including:

Injections: Hormone treatment injections are often administered every few weeks or months and can be administered in the office or clinic of a healthcare professional.

Oral Medications: Hormone therapy pills are taken orally and can be taken daily or on an as-needed basis.

Hormone therapy implants are little pellets that are implanted beneath the skin and steadily release medication over a period of several months.

Hormone therapy is classified into two types:

<u>Agonists of luteinizing hormone-releasing hormone (LHRH):</u> These drugs act by preventing the body from generating testosterone. They are typically administered through injection and can be used alone or in conjunction with other drugs.

<u>Anti-androgens</u>: These drugs function by preventing male hormones from acting on prostate cancer cells. They are commonly given as pills or injections in conjunction with LHRH agonists.

Hormone therapy can be utilized in a variety of circumstances, including:

As the principal treatment for metastatic or advanced prostate cancer. It is used as a neoadjuvant therapy, which means it is administered prior to other therapies such as surgery or radiation therapy in order to reduce the prostate gland and make it easier to remove or treat.

As an adjuvant therapy, it is administered following other therapies such as surgery or radiation therapy to reduce the risk of cancer recurrence.

Side effects of hormone therapy include hot flashes, diminished sex drive, erectile dysfunction, weight gain, and loss as well as muscle mass reduction. Patients should examine the potential risks and advantages of hormone therapy with their healthcare provider, as well as raise any questions they may have. Regular check-ins with healthcare specialists are also necessary to monitor any changes in cancer and adapt the treatment strategy as needed.

Chemotherapy and other methodical treatments

Chemotherapy is a systemic treatment that uses chemicals to kill cancer cells all over the body. Chemotherapy may be used in the treatment of prostate cancer that has progressed to other regions of the body or that is no longer responding to hormone therapy. While chemotherapy can be beneficial in treating prostate cancer, it is rarely utilized as a first-line treatment option and is usually reserved for cases where other treatments have failed. Docetaxel, cabazitaxel, and mitoxantrone are examples of chemotherapy medications that may be used to treat prostate cancer. These medications are typically administered via intravenous (IV) infusion, which means the medication is injected directly into a vein in the arm. Side effects of chemotherapy may include exhaustion, nausea and vomiting, hair loss, and an increased risk of infection.

In addition to chemotherapy, various other systemic treatments for prostate cancer are available, including:

Immunotherapy is a sort of treatment that uses the body's immune system to combat cancer cells. Immune checkpoint inhibitors are a type of immunotherapy that prevents particular proteins in cancer cells from being recognized and attacked by the immune system. Immunotherapy may be used to treat advanced cancer.

Targeted therapy is a sort of treatment that targets certain molecules or proteins that are important in cancer cell proliferation and dissemination. Drugs for targeted therapy may be used in conjunction with other therapies such as chemotherapy or hormone therapy.

Radiopharmaceutical therapy involves the use of radioactive chemicals that can be directed toward cancer cells in the body. These medicines, which can be administered via IV infusion or injection, can assist to kill cancer cells while causing minimal damage to healthy organs.

Patients should examine the potential risks and advantages of these treatments with their healthcare professional, as well as raise any questions they may have. Prostate cancer treatment strategies are often tailored to the patient depending on a variety of factors, aspects such as cancer's stage and grade, the patient's overall health, and their personal preferences. Regular check-ins with healthcare specialists are also necessary to monitor any changes in cancer and adapt the treatment strategy as needed.

IMMUNOTHERAPY AS WELL AS TARGETED THERAPY

Systemic treatments such as immunotherapy and targeted therapy are becoming increasingly significant in the treatment of prostate cancer.

Immunotherapy

Immunotherapy is a sort of treatment that uses the immune system's power to combat cancer cells. Normally, the immune system recognizes and attacks foreign cells and substances in the body, including cancer cells. Cancer cells, on the other hand, are frequently able to avoid identification and attack by the immune system.

Immunotherapy works by either activating or suppressing the immune system to spot and kill cancer cells or by preventing cancer cells from evading the immune system. Immune checkpoint inhibitors are one type of immunotherapy that has been approved for the treatment of advanced prostate cancer. These medications function by inhibiting specific proteins on cancer cells or immune cells that interact with cancer cells, helping the immune system recognize and destroy cancer cells more effectively.

While immunotherapy has shown promise in the treatment of some cancers, such as melanoma and lung cancer, it has proven less beneficial in the treatment of prostate cancer. However, ongoing clinical trials are looking into how immunotherapy can be used in conjunction with other therapies, such as chemotherapy and radiation therapy, to enhance outcomes for individuals with prostate cancer.

Targeted Therapy

Targeted therapy is a sort of treatment that targets specific molecules or proteins involved in cancer cell development and dissemination.

Unlike chemotherapy, which kills rapidly dividing cells, targeted therapy is intended to interfere with specific processes or proteins that are essential for cancer cell survival and proliferation.

Androgen receptor signaling inhibitors are one type of targeted therapy that has been approved for the treatment of advanced prostate cancer. These medications target the androgen receptor, a protein that is essential for the growth and survival of prostate cancer cells. Androgen receptor signaling inhibitors can reduce the proliferation of prostate cancer cells and may assist to postpone disease progression.

Other varieties of targeted medications that target specific mutations or abnormalities in cancer cells, as well as medications that interfere with the tumor microenvironment or blood arteries that give nutrients to the tumor, are among the therapies being studied for the treatment of prostate cancer.

Immunotherapy and targeted therapy, like all cancer treatments, can have substantial side effects. Patients should speak with their healthcare provider about the potential advantages and dangers of these medicines, and engage with their healthcare team to manage any adverse effects that may emerge.

ALTERNATIVE AND COMPLEMENTARY THERAPIES

Patients battling prostate cancer frequently use complementary and alternative therapies to improve their quality of life and control their symptoms. While these treatments may be beneficial for certain Patients with prostate cancer can use them to improve their quality of life and manage their symptoms. While these therapies may be beneficial for some individuals, it is crucial to stress that they are not a replacement for normal medical treatments and should be used in conjunction with them.

Complementary and alternative therapies that patients with prostate cancer may use include:

Acupuncture is the insertion of tiny needles into particular places on the body to promote healing and pain relief. Acupuncture may help relieve symptoms of prostate cancer such as discomfort and exhaustion, according to some research.

Massage Therapy is the manipulation of soft tissue to promote relaxation and relieve muscle tension. It may assist people with prostate cancer manage discomfort and improving their overall quality of life.

Dietary Supplements: Some patients may utilize dietary supplements to improve their general health and well-being, such as vitamins, minerals, and herbal medicines. Patients should be cautious, however, because some of these medications may interfere with traditional cancer treatments or have negative effects of their own.

Mind-body therapies, such as meditation and yoga, may assist people with prostate cancer reduce stress and anxiety. These treatments may also aid in the improvement of sleep and general quality of life.

To ensure that complementary and alternative therapies are safe and successful, patients should discuss their use with their healthcare professionals. Patients must also keep in mind that some of these therapies may not be reimbursed by insurance and may necessitate out-of-pocket costs.

4

LIVING WITH PROSTATE CANCER

How to Handle a Diagnosis

Receiving a prostate cancer diagnosis can be a difficult and emotional event. Coping with the diagnosis and treating the disease's physical and emotional components can be challenging for individuals and their families. This chapter will go over numerous coping tactics for men who have been diagnosed with prostate cancer.

Seek help: Seeking support is one of the most important things a patient can do after being diagnosed with prostate cancer. This can take various forms, including family and friend support, support groups, and counseling. Support groups and therapy can be especially beneficial for people who are having difficulty accepting their diagnosis or are suffering substantial emotional hardship.

Inform yourself: Knowledge is power, and learning more about prostate cancer might make you feel less anxious and uncertain. Patients should consult their doctors and conduct their own research to understand more about the disease, treatment options, and what to expect.

Communicate honestly: It is critical for patients to communicate openly about their sentiments and concerns with their healthcare providers and family members. Patients should also be honest with themselves about how they feel and seek help if they are experiencing emotional difficulties.

Change your lifestyle: Making lifestyle adjustments, such as altering your food and exercising more, can help enhance your general health and well-being. Patients with prostate cancer may benefit from a diet rich in fruits, vegetables, and whole grains and low in saturated fat from processed foods and red meat. Exercise can also help relieve stress and anxiety while improving the overall quality of life.

Manage the side effects of treatment: Prostate cancer therapies can result in a variety of physical and mental side effects, including fatigue, discomfort, and sexual dysfunction. Patients should collaborate closely with their healthcare professionals to manage these side effects and create coping mechanisms for any physical or mental difficulties that arise.

Have a positive attitude: It might be difficult to have a good attitude when coping with a serious illness like prostate cancer, but it can help to minimize stress and worry and enhance the overall quality of life. Patients should concentrate on what they can manage and look for methods to stay engaged and active in their lives.

Explore complementary therapies such as acupuncture and massage therapy can assist patients with prostate cancer manage their symptoms and improving their quality of life. Patients should consult with their healthcare physician before using complementary therapies to confirm that they are safe and effective.

Coping with a prostate cancer diagnosis can be difficult, but there are several ways that patients can take to manage the physical and emotional elements of the disease. Seeking help, educating yourself, communicating freely, changing your lifestyle, managing treatment side effects, being positive, and investigating complementary therapies can all help you cope with a prostate cancer diagnosis.

Patients should collaborate closely with their healthcare providers to design a treatment plan, a thorough approach for managing the disease and increasing the overall quality of life.

Managing Side Effects of Treatment

Treatment for prostate cancer can have a variety of physical and mental side effects that might have an influence on a patient's quality of life. Managing these side effects is a critical element of prostate cancer treatment, and patients should collaborate with their healthcare professionals to establish coping techniques for any physical or emotional difficulties that arise.

Fatigue is a typical side effect of prostate cancer treatment that can be difficult for patients to manage. Patients should attempt to get enough rest in order to overcome fatigue, but they should also engage in regular physical activity, such as walking or swimming, which can help to boost energy levels. Patients should also strive to eat a balanced diet and avoid coffee and alcohol, both of which can cause weariness.

Discomfort and pain: Treatment for prostate cancer can cause discomfort, particularly in the lower back, hips, and pelvic area. Patients should share any pain they are feeling with their healthcare provider, who may advise them on over-the-counter or prescription pain medications, as well as other pain management options such as physical therapy or acupuncture.

Sexual dysfunction: Prostate cancer treatment can result in sexual dysfunction, such as erectile dysfunction and libido loss. Patients should address these side effects with their doctor, who may prescribe medicine such as sildenafil (Viagra) or other treatments such as penile injections or vacuum devices. Patients may also benefit from counseling or support groups to assist them in coping with their condition and the emotional impact of sexual dysfunction.

Incontinence: A typical side effect of prostate cancer treatment is incontinence, or the inability to regulate urinating. Patients should collaborate closely with their healthcare practitioner to manage this side effect, which may involve pelvic muscle-strengthening activities such as Kegel exercises or medication to minimize bladder spasms.

Prostate cancer treatment might result in gastrointestinal issues such as diarrhea and constipation. Patients should address these adverse effects with their healthcare provider, who may propose dietary or pharmaceutical adjustments to alleviate the symptoms.

Hot flashes can be caused by hormone therapy, which is a typical treatment for prostate cancer. Patients should address these adverse effects with their healthcare provider, who may advise them to take medication, such as venlafaxine (Effexor), or to try other methods Acupuncture, for example, can be used to manage these symptoms.

Anxiety and despair: Because prostate cancer therapy can be emotionally draining, patients may feel anxiety or depression. Patients should address any emotional symptoms they are having with their healthcare provider, who may advise them to seek therapy, join support groups, or take medication to alleviate these symptoms.

Lymphedema: Lymphedema, or swelling in the legs or feet, can result from prostate cancer surgery or radiation therapy. Patients should collaborate closely with their healthcare practitioner to manage this side effect, which may involve lymphatic drainage exercises or the use of compression garments.

Changes in cognition: Prostate cancer treatment might result in cognitive changes such as trouble concentrating or memory loss, patients should address these adverse effects with their healthcare physician, who may offer coping tactics such as writing things down or using memory aides.

Chemotherapy can cause peripheral neuropathy, which is characterized by numbness or tingling in the hands or feet. Patients should address these side effects with their doctor, who may provide medicine, such as gabapentin (Neurontin), or other treatments, such as physical therapy, to alleviate these problems.

Treating the adverse effects of prostate cancer treatment is an important element of care for prostate cancer patients. Patients should collaborate closely with their healthcare professionals to create coping techniques for any physical or mental issues that may arise. Medication, physical therapy, counseling, and support may be used as strategies.

Medication, physical therapy, counseling, support groups, or lifestyle modifications like exercise and a balanced diet may be used as strategies.

Interaction with medical professionals

Communication with healthcare experts is critical in the treatment of prostate cancer. It can assist patients in comprehending their diagnosis, treatment options, and potential adverse effects. Effective communication can also assist patients in receiving appropriate care and assistance, as well as improving their overall quality of life.

Communication with healthcare providers has various advantages

Grasp the diagnosis: Patients with prostate cancer who interact well with their healthcare professionals will have a better grasp of their diagnosis. Understanding the stage of cancer, treatment options, and potential side effects are all part of this.

Access to adequate care: Communication with healthcare practitioners can assist patients in receiving proper care, this involves prompt access to diagnostic tests, treatment, and care.

Adherence to treatment programs can be improved by effective communication with healthcare practitioners. Patients who understand their treatment plan will be more inclined to stick to it.

Improved quality of life: Prostate cancer patients who communicate with their healthcare professionals can better manage their symptoms and side effects. It can also assist patients in meeting their emotional and psychological demands, thereby improving their overall quality of life.

Patients who interact effectively with their healthcare providers have a higher chance of having excellent health results. This includes increased survival rates, fewer hospitalizations, and better general health. Prostate cancer patients must communicate openly and honestly with their healthcare providers. Patients should be prepared to ask inquiries and share their concerns. Patients can get information from healthcare providers regarding their diagnosis, treatment options, and potential adverse effects. They can also assist patients in managing their symptoms and side effects, as well as addressing any emotional or psychological issues.

Patients can benefit from maintaining a record of their symptoms and side effects in addition to discussing them with healthcare experts. This can assist patients understand their illness and provide valuable information to healthcare practitioners regarding their treatment.

Prostate cancer sufferers must communicate effectively with their healthcare providers. It can assist patients in better understanding their diagnosis, receiving appropriate care, adhering to treatment programs, and improving their quality of life as well as improving health outcomes. Patients should interact with their healthcare professionals openly and honestly, and they should be prepared to ask questions and share any concerns they may have.

ASSISTANCE FOR PATIENTS AND CAREGIVERS

Prostate cancer can be a difficult diagnosis for both sufferers and their caretakers. Patients and caregivers may require assistance throughout the cancer journey, from diagnosis to treatment and beyond. Patients and caregivers can get a variety of sorts of assistance, including:

Medical Assistance: Patients with prostate cancer require medical assistance from healthcare providers. Access to diagnostic testing, therapy, and support services are all part of this. Healthcare providers can assist patients in managing their symptoms and side effects, as well as dealing with any emotional or psychological issues.

Emotional Support: Patients and caregivers dealing with prostate cancer may face emotional difficulties. Counseling, support groups, and individual therapy can all provide emotional support. These materials can assist patients and carers in dealing with the emotional consequences of prostate cancer.

Practical Assistance: Patients and carers may require practical assistance to handle daily duties. This can include help with housework, transportation, and meal preparation.

Financial Assistance: Cancer treatment can be expensive, and patients and carers may seek assistance. Access to insurance coverage, financial aid programs, and assistance in negotiating insurance and financial challenges are all examples of financial assistance.

Patients and caregivers with prostate cancer may require education and information on the diagnosis, treatment options, and side effects. Education and information can be beneficial. Healthcare providers, support groups, and online resources are all available.

Palliative Care is a type of care that focuses on treating symptoms and enhancing the quality of life for people suffering from serious illnesses such as cancer. Palliative care can be administered at any stage of prostate cancer and can assist patients and carers in coping with the disease's physical, emotional, and spiritual burdens.

Survivorship Support: After treatment has concluded, survivorship support focuses on the physical, emotional, and practical needs of patients and carers. Follow-up treatment, access to support groups, and education and information regarding long-term side effects and ongoing health maintenance are all examples of survivor support.

There are numerous sorts of support accessible to prostate cancer patients and carers. Medical, emotional, practical, budgetary considerations, education and information, palliative care, and survivor support are all valuable services that can assist patients and families in coping with the problems of prostate cancer. Patients and caregivers must be aware of these services and have access to the support they require throughout their cancer experience.

Other non-medical assistance for prostate patients includes...

Numerous non-medical services can help prostate cancer patients manage their disease and improve their general well-being, in addition to medical and healthcare support.

These are some examples:

Social support: Patients might tremendously benefit from the assistance of friends and family members. Social support can help patients cope emotionally with their diagnosis and treatment, as well as give practical assistance with everyday duties.

Exercise and physical exercise can assist prostate cancer patients manage symptoms and side effects such as fatigue, discomfort, and muscle mass loss. Exercise has also been demonstrated to improve the overall quality of life and lower the likelihood of recurrence.

Nutritional support: good nutrition is crucial for prostate cancer patients since it can help manage the side effects of treatment and enhance overall health. Working with a nutritionist or dietitian to design a healthy eating plan may benefit patients

.

Alternative therapies, such as acupuncture, massage, and yoga, may help some individuals find respite from their symptoms. Before pursuing these choices, patients should consult with their healthcare professionals.

Patients may benefit from spiritual and emotional assistance.

Meditation or prayer can provide spiritual or emotional support. These strategies can help cancer patients manage stress, anxiety, and other emotional issues.

As previously stated, the expense of cancer treatment can be high, and patients may require financial assistance. Access to financial assistance programs, guidance with insurance and financial concerns, and assistance with medical costs are examples of non-medical support.

Patients may benefit from joining a prostate cancer support group, where they can connect with others who are going through similar situations. Prostate cancer advocacy organizations can also give information and resources about prostate cancer research, activism, and public policy.

Non-medical assistance can play a significant role in assisting prostate cancer patients in managing their illnesses and boosting their general well-being. Patients can obtain vital services such as social support, exercise and physical activity, dietary support, alternative therapies, spiritual and emotional support, financial support, and advocacy and support groups to aid them through their cancer experience.

CHANGES IN LIFESTYLE TO REDUCE RISK AND IMPROVE OUTCOMES

Several lifestyle adjustments may help minimize the risk of acquiring prostate cancer or improve results for those who have already been diagnosed. These are some examples:

A Nutritious Diet rich in fruits, vegetables, whole grains, and lean protein may help lower the chance of developing prostate cancer. It is also critical to minimize your consumption of red meat and processed meals.

Exercise Regularly: Physical activity regularly may help minimize the chance of developing prostate cancer, as well as improve results for individuals who have already been diagnosed. Exercise can also aid in the management of treatment-related side effects such as fatigue, as well as enhance overall quality of life.

Maintaining a Healthy Weight: Being overweight or obese increases the chance of developing prostate cancer and worsens the prognosis for those who have been diagnosed. Maintaining a healthy weight through diet and exercise may aid in lowering this risk.

Quitting Smoking: Smoking has been related to an increased risk of prostate cancer as well as other types of cancer. Smoking cessation can help lower this risk and improve overall health outcomes.

Limiting Alcohol Consumption: Drinking too much alcohol has been related to an increased risk of getting prostate cancer. Limiting alcohol consumption may assist to lessen this risk.

Adjusting to these lifestyle adjustments can be difficult, but they are doable with the correct help and resources. Working with a healthcare provider or a qualified dietitian to design a healthy food plan or exercise routine may assist patients. Patients who are having difficulty making these lifestyle adjustments may benefit from support groups and counseling.

Furthermore, by participating in healthy activities together and supporting healthy behaviors, family and friends can create a supportive environment.

It is important to remember that lifestyle changes require time and effort, but the rewards can be substantial in terms of lowering the chance of acquiring prostate cancer or improving outcomes for those who have been diagnosed

5

PREVENTION AND NEXT STEPS

Preventive Measures and Screening Guidelines

Prostate cancer management begins with prevention. While there is no sure strategy to avoid prostate cancer, there are many steps that can be taken to minimize the risk. These steps are as follows:

Men over the age of 50 should get frequent check-ups with their healthcare practitioner, which should include a prostate exam and a PSA blood test. Men who have a family history of prostate cancer or are at a higher risk of developing the disease should begin screening at a younger age.

Maintaining a healthy lifestyle, as previously stated, can help minimize the risk of acquiring prostate cancer through nutrition, exercise, and weight control.

Consider Chemoprevention: chemoprevention entails using medications or other substances to prevent the development of cancer. Some drugs, such as finasteride and dutasteride, have been found to lessen the incidence of prostate cancer in men who are predisposed to it.

Understand your Family History: Men with a family history of prostate cancer may be more likely to develop the disease. It is critical to discuss your family history with your healthcare professional, as well as proper screening and prevention steps.

Avoid Environmental Toxins: Certain environmental toxins, such as pesticides and industrial chemicals, may raise the chance of getting prostate cancer. Using protective equipment or choosing organic items to prevent these chemicals may help lessen the risk.

Guidelines for screening Prostate cancer have sparked much debate and controversy, *the American Cancer Society* recommends that men discuss the risks and benefits of prostate cancer screening with their healthcare provider beginning at age 50 for most men, or at age 45 for men at higher risk (such as African American men or men with a family history of prostate cancer). Screening should be decided depending on an individual's unique preferences and risk factors.

A prostate-specific antigen (PSA) blood test and a digital rectal exam (DRE) are generally used in screening. PSA levels that are elevated may indicate the existence of prostate cancer, but more testing is required to confirm a diagnosis.

It is critical to recognize that screening has limitations and may lead to false positives or overdiagnosis, resulting in needless therapies and unwanted effects. Men should consider the potential risks and advantages of screening with their healthcare physician before making an informed decision based on their unique situation.

Prevention and early detection are critical in the treatment of prostate cancer. Maintaining a healthy lifestyle, contemplating chemoprevention, understanding your family history, avoiding environmental pollutants, and adhering to suitable screening standards can all help minimize your risk of developing prostate cancer or identify it at an early stage when it is most treatable.

ADVANCES IN PROSTATE CANCER RESEARCH, FUTURE THERAPY, AND PREVENTION TECHNIQUES

Prostate cancer research has improved dramatically in recent years, yielding fresh insights into the disease's biology, about the disease, as well as novel techniques for prevention, diagnosis, and therapy. The following are some of the most promising advancements in prostate cancer research:

Precision medicine entails adapting treatment to an individual's unique genetic profile as well as the characteristics of their malignancy. This method can help to increase therapeutic effectiveness while avoiding negative effects. Precision medicine has resulted in the development of novel medications that target specific genetic abnormalities or other biomarkers in prostate cancer.

Immunotherapy is the use of the body's own immune system to target and destroy cancer cells. Immunotherapy has shown promise in early-stage trials for prostate cancer, with some patients reporting considerable tumor shrinking and better survival.

Liquid biopsies are tests that evaluate tumor DNA in liquid form before it is sucked into circulation. Liquid biopsies are less intrusive and less time-consuming than standard tissue biopsies, and they can provide real-time information on disease progression.

Artificial intelligence (AI) and machine learning are being used to analyze enormous volumes of data and uncover patterns that may be useful for predicting prostate cancer risk, early detection of the disease, and therapy optimization.

Researchers have been able to discover genetic changes that may raise the chance of developing prostate cancer thanks to advances in genetic testing. This information can be used to guide screening and preventative initiatives.

Minimally invasive treatments: As an alternative to surgery and radiation therapy, minimally invasive treatments such as focal therapy and high-intensity focused ultrasound (HIFU) are being developed. These treatments may be less intrusive, have shorter recovery times, and have fewer adverse effects.

Overall, developments in prostate cancer research hold significant potential for bettering the disease's results for patients. More study, however, is required to completely comprehend the biology of prostate cancer and develop more effective prevention, detection, and treatment options.

TREATMENT AND PREVENTION STRATEGIES FOR THE FUTURE

With nearly 1.4 million cases worldwide in 2020, prostate cancer is the most commonly diagnosed cancer in men. Prostate cancer remains a major public health concern, despite breakthroughs in screening and treatment. As researchers continue to understand more about the biology of the illness, new prospects for prostate cancer prevention and treatment emerge.

a. **Combination Treatments**: Combination treatments are a new field of treatment for prostate cancer. Researchers seek to get better results than single-agent therapy by combining several medications or treatment techniques. Combining radiation therapy with immunotherapy or hormone therapy, for example, may assist to stimulate the immune system's response to cancer cells and improve treatment effectiveness.

b. **Gene Editing**: CRISPR-Cas9 gene editing techniques are being investigated as potential therapeutics for prostate cancer. These methods enable researchers to alter the DNA of cancer cells in order to make them more susceptible to existing treatments or to induce programmed cell death.

c. **Nanotechnology**: Nanoparticles are being developed and designed as a technique of delivering medications directly to cancer cells. This strategy may assist to reduce adverse effects and increase therapeutic efficacy.

d.   **Therapies   Targeting   Prostate-Specific Membrane Antigen** (PSMA): PSMA-targeted therapies are a novel class of medications that specifically target the PSMA protein, which is abundant in prostate cancer cells. These medications can be utilized to directly deliver radioactive isotopes or chemotherapeutic chemicals to cancer cells while causing minimal damage to healthy tissue.

MEDICAL PRECISION

Precision medicine is adapting treatment to an individual's unique genetic profile as well as tumor features. This method can help to increase therapeutic effectiveness while avoiding negative effects.

a. **Genomic Profiling**: Genomic profiling is evaluating a patient's tumor for genetic alterations or other biomarkers that may be the present cause of cancer. This data can be used to guide treatment decisions and uncover novel therapeutic targets.

b. **Liquid Biopsies**: Liquid biopsies are a non-invasive method of testing tumor DNA in the bloodstream. This method can provide real-time information on illness progression and assist guide treatment decisions.

c. **Imaging Techniques**: Advances in imaging techniques such as positron emission tomography (PET) and magnetic resonance imaging (MRI) are allowing doctors to detect and monitor prostate cancer with greater accuracy. These strategies can also be used to guide treatment decisions and track therapeutic efficacy.

NEW SCREENING TECHNIQUES

Screening for prostate cancer is contentious because the benefits of early detection must be balanced against the risks of overdiagnosis as well as abuse. New screening methods, on the other hand, are being developed that may increase the accuracy of prostate cancer detection while reducing the need for intrusive treatments.

a. **Biomarkers**: Biomarkers are chemicals or genetic markers that can be used to diagnose cancer. Several biomarkers, including prostate-specific antigen (PSA), assays that are more specific and sensitive than current tests, are being developed for use in prostate cancer screening.

b. **Imaging Methods**: Advances in imaging methods are also being used to screen for prostate cancer. Multiparametric MRI (mpMRI), for example, can be used to detect worrisome lesions in the prostate, eliminating the need for invasive biopsies.

PREVENTION

Prostate cancer prevention is a key focus of scientific efforts. Several techniques are being investigated for their ability to minimize the chance of acquiring prostate cancer or decrease the advancement of the disease.

- ***Lifestyle Modifications***

Lifestyle factors such as food and exercise may influence prostate cancer risk. Consuming a balanced diet reduced in red and processed meats and consuming a diet low in red and processed meats is one of the main lifestyle modifications that can help lower the risk of developing prostate cancer and improve outcomes for those who have already been diagnosed is eating foods high in fruits, vegetables, and whole grains. A diet strong in animal fats and red meat has been found in studies to raise the risk of prostate cancer, whereas a diet rich in fruits and vegetables, particularly those high in lycopene and selenium, can help lower the risk.

Lycopene is an antioxidant that can be found in tomatoes, watermelon, and pink grapefruit. Men who consume more lycopene had a lower risk of acquiring prostate cancer, according to research. Selenium is a mineral found in nuts, fish, and whole grains that has anti-cancer properties.

Regular exercise, in addition to a balanced diet, can help lower the risk of prostate cancer and improve outcomes for those who have been diagnosed. Men who engage in regular physical activity had a lower risk of acquiring prostate cancer and may have better results after treatment, according to research.

Maintaining a healthy weight, eliminating smoking, and limiting alcohol use are other lifestyle modifications that can reduce prostate cancer

While making these lifestyle adjustments might be difficult, there are numerous tools available to assist men and their families in adapting to these changes. Healthcare practitioners, dietitians, and exercise specialists can all help you make these lifestyle adjustments. Support groups can also be a great resource for men and their families who have been diagnosed with prostate cancer and are looking for strategies to cope with the disease's physical and emotional burdens.

CONCLUSION

prostate cancer is a major health problem for men, and early detection and treatment can make a big difference in results. To guarantee timely discovery, men must grasp the risk factors, symptoms, and diagnostic techniques involved in prostate cancer. help minimize the risk of prostate cancer ensuring that patients receive the assistance they require. Support groups and other resources can be extremely helpful in offering emotional support and practical information to men and their families dealing with a prostate cancer diagnosis.

Raising prostate cancer awareness is critical for early identification and adequate treatment. Men should take charge of their health and collaborate with their doctors to ensure they undergo the necessary screening and diagnostic procedures. While prostate cancer is a difficult diagnosis to face, there is hope, and with the correct therapy and support, men may conquer the disease and live healthy, fulfilling lives.